A WHOLESALE PERSPECTIVE OF INFERTILITY

Infertility Remedy in male and female.

Elizabeth R Smith.

Table of contents

Chapter 1

A wholesale perspective of infertility.

Up to 15% of couples experience infertility, which is defined as failure to conceive within 12 months of unprotected sexual activity or therapeutic donor insemination in women under 35, or within 6 months in women over 35. Any patient who is infertile by definition or has a high risk of becoming infertile may be given an infertility evaluation. If clinically necessary, women over the age of 35 should undergo treatment and an expedited evaluation after six months of unsuccessful pregnancy attempts. More immediate evaluation and treatment are necessary for women over the age of 40. A woman should receive an immediate evaluation from the obstetrician-gynecologist if she has a condition that is known to contribute to infertility. An initial workup's crucial elements include a review of the physical exam, medical history, and any additional tests recommended. Tests on the female partner will concentrate on structural abnormalities, ovarian reserve, and ovulatory function. Imaging the reproductive system can reveal important details about ailments that affect fertility. Imaging techniques can evaluate ovarian reserve, find pelvic pathology, and check tubal patency. In 40–50% of couples, the male factor is the cause of infertility. A basic medical history and evaluation of the male partner are necessary right away due to the high prevalence of male Factors in infertile heterosexual couples. It is reasonable for a woman's health expert to request the partner's medical history and order the semen analysis. Additionally, it makes sense to refer all men experiencing infertility to a physician who specializes in male reproductive medicine. Up to 30% of infertile couples may have an undiagnosed infertility diagnosis. These patients should, at the very least, exhibit signs of ovulation, tubal patency, and a normal semen analysis.

Recommendations and Conclusions

The following conclusions and recommendations are made by the American Society for Reproductive Medicine (ASRM) and the American College of Obstetricians and Gynecologists (ACOG):

- Any patient who is infertile by definition or has a high risk of becoming infertile may be given an infertility evaluation.

- If clinically necessary, women over the age of 35 should undergo treatment and an expedited evaluation after six months of unsuccessful pregnancy attempts. More immediate evaluation and treatment are necessary for women over the age of 40. A woman should receive an immediate evaluation from the obstetrician-gynecologist if she has a condition that is known to contribute to infertility.
- If there is a partner, they should be asked for a thorough medical history that includes information pertinent to any potential etiologies of infertility.

- The female partner should undergo a targeted physical examination that focuses on vital signs and includes a thyroid, breast, and pelvic examination.

- Tests on the female partner will concentrate on structural abnormalities, ovarian reserve, and ovulatory function.

- Imaging the reproductive system can reveal important details about ailments that affect fertility. Imaging techniques can evaluate ovarian reserve, find pelvic pathology, and check tubal patency.

- It is reasonable for a woman's health expert to request the partner's medical history and order the semen analysis. As an alternative, it makes sense to refer all men experiencing infertility to a qualified healthcare professional with experience in treating male reproductive issues.

Chapter 2

Main causes of infertility in women

1. Lack of ovulation.
   Failure to ovulate, which affects 40% of women with infertility problems, is the most typical overall cause of female infertility.

   1 Numerous factors can prevent ovulation, including:

   gynecological or ovarian disorders like polycystic ovary syndrome (PCOS) or primary ovarian insufficiency (POI) (PCOS)

   Aging, including "diminished ovarian reserve," describes a woman's ovary's low egg production as a result of natural aging.

   Endocrine disorders affect how much or how little of a hormone or group of hormones the body produces.

Examples include thyroid disease and issues with the hypothalamus.

2. Menstrual cycle issues.
    Infertility can result from issues with the menstrual cycle, which prepares the female body for pregnancy. The menstrual cycle has several phases, and issues with any one of them can make it difficult or impossible to conceive.

3. Menstrual disorders include:

    Dysmenorrhea is the term for uncomfortable cramps. Premenstrual syndrome is the term used to describe the physical and mental symptoms that appear before menstruation. Heavy bleeding, such as protracted menstrual periods or excessive bleeding during a period of normal length, is referred to as menorrhagia.

4. Issues with the reproductive system's structure.

The presence of abnormal tissue in the uterus or fallopian tubes is a common symptom of structural issues.

Eggs cannot travel from the ovaries to the uterus and sperm cannot reach the uterus if the fallopian tubes are blocked unable to penetrate the egg to fertilize it. Infertility can also result from uterine structural issues, such as those that could prevent implantation. Some specific structural problems that can cause infertility include:

Endometriosis is when tissue that normally lines the inside of the uterus is found in other places, such as blocking the fallopian tubes
Uterine fibroids are growths that appear within and around the wall of the uterus, although most women with

fibroids do not have problems with fertility and can get pregnant. However, some women with fibroids may not be able to get pregnant naturally or may have multiple miscarriages or preterm labor.

Polyps are noncancerous growths on the inside surface of the uterus. Polyps can interfere with the function of the uterus and make it difficult for a woman to remain pregnant after conception. Surgical removal of the polyps can increase the chances for a woman to get pregnant.

Scarring in the uterus from previous injuries, infections, or surgery. Scarring may increase the risk of miscarriage and may interfere with implantation, thus leading to infertility.

An unusually shaped uterus, can affect implantation and the ability to carry a pregnancy to term.

5. Infections. ...
Infections can also cause infertility in men and women.

Untreated gonorrhea and chlamydia in women can lead to pelvic inflammatory disease, which might cause scarring that blocks the fallopian tubes. Untreated syphilis increases the risk of a pregnant woman having a stillbirth. More information about infections that may affect fertility can be found on the sexually transmitted infections (STIs) health topic page.

Chronic infections in the cervix and surgical treatment of cervical lesions associated with human papillomavirus (HPV) infection can also reduce the amount or quality of cervical mucus. Problems with this sticky or slippery substance that collects on the cervix and in the vagina can make it difficult for women to get pregnant.1

The Centers for Disease Control and Prevention recommends that all boys and girls age 11 or 12 be vaccinated against HPV. Men and women who weren't vaccinated as preteens can also get the vaccine into their early to mid-20s.

Failure of an Egg to Mature Properly.
...
Eggs may not mature properly for a variety of reasons, ranging from conditions such as PCOS to obesity to a lack of specific proteins needed for the egg to mature.

An immature egg may not be released at the correct time, may not make it down the fallopian tubes, or may not be able to be fertilized

6. Implantation Failure. ...

Implantation failure refers to the failure of a fertilized egg to implant in the uterine wall to begin pregnancy. While the specific cause of implantation failure is often unknown, possibilities include:

- Genetic defects in the embryo
- Thin endometrium (pronounced en-doh-MEE-tree-uhm)
- Embryonic defects
- Endometriosis
- Progesterone resistance
- Scar tissue in the endometrial cavity

Endometriosis. ...
Endometriosis occurs when the cells that normally line the uterine cavity, called the endometrium, are found outside the uterus instead. A more detailed description of endometriosis can be found on the NICHD endometriosis topic page.

Research has found a link between infertility and endometriosis. Studies show that between 25% and 50% of infertile women have endometriosis and between 30% and 40% of women with endometriosis are infertile.6,7,8 Scientists do not know the exact cause of infertility in women with endometriosis.

Current theories on how endometriosis causes infertility include the following:

Changes in the structure of the female reproductive organs may occur. Endometriosis can cause pelvic adhesions made of scar tissue to form between nearby structures, such as between the ovary and pelvic wall. This can obstruct and affect the release of the egg after ovulation. Scarring in the fallopian tube can interrupt or block the egg's movement through the fallopian tube. The lining of the abdomen, which is called the peritoneum (pronounced pair-ih-tuh-NEE-uhm), may go through changes that affect its function:

In women with endometriosis, the amount of fluid inside the peritoneum often increases.
The fluid in the peritoneum contains substances that can negatively affect the functions of the egg, sperm, and fallopian tubes.
Chemical changes in the lining of the uterus that occur as a result of endometriosis may affect an embryo's ability to implant properly and make it difficult for a woman to stay pregnant after conception.

7. Polycystic Ovary Syndrome (PCOS)
   PCOS is one of the most common causes of female infertility.9 It is a condition in which a woman's ovaries and, in some cases, adrenal glands produce more androgens (a type of hormone) than normal. High levels of these hormones interfere with the development of ovarian follicles and the release of eggs during ovulation. As a result, fluid-filled sacs, or cysts,

can develop within the ovaries. A more detailed description can be found on the NICHD PCOS topic page.

Researchers estimate that 5% to 10% of women in the United States have PCOS.10 The exact cause of PCOS is unknown, but current research suggests that a combination of genetic and environmental factors leads to the disease.

Uterine Fibroids
Uterine fibroids are noncancerous growths that form inside the uterus. Uterine fibroids can cause symptoms in some cases, depending on their size and location. Scientists do not know what causes fibroids to form, but it is believed that there may be a genetic basis.

Fibroids can contribute to infertility and are found in 5% to 10% of infertile women.12 Fibroids located in the uterine cavity (as opposed to those that grow within the uterine wall) or those that are larger than 6 centimeters in diameter are more likely to have a negative effect on fertility. Fibroids are more likely to affect a woman's fertility if they

Change the position of the cervix, which can reduce the number of sperm that enter the uterus
Change the shape of the uterus, which can interfere with the movement of sperm or implantation
Block the fallopian tubes, which prevents sperm from reaching the egg and keeps a fertilized egg from moving to the uterus
Interfere with blood flow to the uterus, which can prevent the embryo from implanting
A more detailed description of uterine fibroids can be found on the NICHD.

Chapter 3

Main causes of infertility in men

These may include:

1. Abnormal sperm production or function due to undescended testicles, genetic defects, health problems such as diabetes, or infections such as chlamydia, gonorrhea, mumps, or HIV. Enlarged veins in the testes (varicocele) also can affect the quality of sperm.

2. Problems with the delivery of sperm due to sexual problems, such as premature ejaculation; certain genetic diseases, such as cystic fibrosis; structural problems, such as a blockage in the testicle; or damage or injury to the reproductive organs.

3. Overexposure to certain environmental factors, such as pesticides and other chemicals, and radiation. Cigarette smoking, alcohol, marijuana, anabolic steroids, and taking medications to treat bacterial infections, high blood pressure, and depression also can affect fertility. Frequent exposure to heat, such as in saunas or hot tubs, can raise body temperature and may affect sperm production.

4. Damage related to cancer and its treatment, including radiation or chemotherapy. Treatment for cancer can impair sperm production, sometimes severely.

Chapter 4

Symptoms of infertility

Common Signs of Infertility in Women.

1. Irregular periods
The average woman's cycle is 28 days long. But anything within a few days of that can be considered normal, as long as those cycles are consistent. For example, a woman who has a 33-day cycle one month, a 31-day cycle the next, and a 35-day cycle after that, is probably having "normal" periods.

But a woman whose cycles vary so greatly that she can't even begin to estimate when her period might arrive is experiencing irregular periods. This can be related to hormone issues, or to polycystic ovarian syndrome (PCOS). Both of these can contribute to infertility.

2. Painful or heavy periods
Most women experience cramps during their periods. But painful periods that interfere with your daily life may be a symptom of endometriosis.

3. No periods
It's not uncommon for women to have an off month here and there. Factors like stress or heavy workouts can cause your period to temporarily disappear. But if you haven't had a period in months, it's time to get your fertility checked.

4.Symptoms of hormone fluctuations
Signs of hormone fluctuations in women could indicate potential issues with fertility. Talk to your doctor if you experience the following:

- skin issues
- reduced sex drive
- facial hair growth
- thinning hair
- weight gain

5. Pain during sex
Some women have experienced painful sex their entire lives, so they've convinced themselves it's normal. But it's not. It could be related to hormone issues, endometriosis, or to other underlying conditions that could also be contributing to infertility.

Common Signs of Infertility in Men

Changes in sexual desire
A man's fertility is also linked to his hormone health. Changes in virility, often governed by hormones, could indicate issues with fertility.

Testicle pain or swelling

There are several different conditions that could lead to pain or swelling in the testicles, many of which could contribute to infertility.

Problems maintaining erection
A man's ability to maintain an erection is often linked to his hormone levels. Reduced hormones may result, which could potentially translate into trouble conceiving.

Issues with ejaculation
Similarly, an inability to ejaculate is a sign that it might be time to visit a doctor.

tiny, solid testicles
In order for a man to be fertile, the health of his testicles is essential. A doctor should investigate any potential problems that could be indicated by small or firm testicles.

The Lesson

An estimated 15 to 20 percent of couples who are trying to get pregnant will experience infertility issues. Infertility due to female factors typically accounts for 40% of problems, whereas infertility due to male factors accounts for 30% to 40% of problems. 20 to 30 percent of the time, a combination of these factors results in infertility.

You're not alone if you've been told you're infertile or think you might have trouble getting pregnant in the future. The medical sector is constantly developing in this area.

Chapter 5

What Are the Treatments for Infertility?

In men, fertility is treated with:

1. Surgery, if the cause is a varicocele (widening of the veins in the scrotum) or a blockage in the vas deferens, tubes that carry sperm.
2. Antibiotics treat infections in the reproductive organs.
3. Medications and counseling to treat problems with erections or ejaculation.
4. Hormone treatments if the problem is a low or high level of certain hormones.

In women, infertility is treated with:

1. hormones and medications for infertility to assist the woman in

ovulating or to replenish hormone levels

2. surgery to open a blocked fallopian tube or remove tissue that is preventing fertility (such as endometriosis).

3. Assisted reproductive technology, or ART, can also be used to treat infertility in both men and women. There are several types of ART:

4. IUI (intrauterine insemination): While a woman is ovulating, sperm is collected and placed inside her uterus.

5. In vitro fertilization (IVF): The sperm and egg are gathered and combined in a laboratory. The fertilized egg takes 3 to 5 days to develop. The embryo is then inserted into the female uterus.

6. The sperm and egg are gathered and quickly inserted into a fallopian tube in GIFT (gamete intrafallopian transfer) and ZIFT (zygote

intrafallopian transfer). With GIFT, the fallopian tube is filled with both sperm and eggs. With ZIFT, the sperm and eggs are combined in a lab, and after 24 hours, a fertilized egg is put into the tube.

www.ingramcontent.com/pod-product-compliance
Lightning Source LLC
Chambersburg PA
CBHW051726250726
48653CB00008B/3221